CANCER DIET
RECIPES FOR
DOGS

**Tested and Trusted Homemade
Meals for Dogs Battling Cancer**

Jeffrey D. Mike

Contents

INTRODUCTION

Grace found herself in the bustling digital age on a mission to support her beloved dog Bella, who was heroically fighting cancer.

Grace determined to pursue every option, sought advice from the broad online world.

She discovered a hidden gem after long research: a comprehensive book of Tested and Trusted homemade dishes specifically developed for pets suffering cancer.

Grace eagerly ordered the book, its pages packed with helpful information. She delved into its pages, uncovering a wealth of healthy nutrients and excellent meal plan.

Grace entered her kitchen with increased confidence, armed with the book's recipes. She thoughtfully prepared meals with broccoli, carrots, blueberries, and sweet potatoes—ingredients known to boost wellbeing and immune system strength.

Grace observed an amazing shift as Bella savored each scrumptious bite. Bella's energy level increased, and she regained her enthusiasm for life.

Grace and Bella paved a path toward hope, health, and shared triumph over cancer thanks to the power of information and cooked food.

Introducing a ray of light for dog owners facing the onerous task of caring for cancer-stricken pets—tested and trusted Homemade Recipes Designed to Support Their Well-Being.

There is solace in knowing that healthy meals can play an important part in bolstering a dog's immune system and providing the power needed to fight this terrible disease.

This book delves into the world of homemade foods designed exclusively for cancer-stricken pets.

Lean proteins like chicken and fish, combined with a variety of vivid veggies and antioxidant-rich fruits, serve as the foundation for these nutritional concoctions.

Every recipe is meticulously crafted with love and attention, ensuring a balance of flavors and essential nutrients.

We embark on a journey to empower dog owners with the knowledge to create simple, yet profoundly beneficial meals for their beloved companions.

Together, let us navigate this path of hope, healing, and a renewed zest for life.

RECIPES

CHICKEN AND RICE DELIGHT

Ingredients

- Cooked chicken breast (1 cup)
- Cooked brown rice (1/2 cup)
- Steamed broccoli (1/2 cup)

Preparation

- Shred the cooked chicken breast.
- Mix the shredded chicken with cooked brown rice and steamed broccoli.
- Serve after cooling.

TURKEY MEATBALLS

Ingredients

- Ground turkey (1/2 pound)
- Grated carrots (1/4 cup)
- Oats (1/4 cup)
- Turmeric (1/4 teaspoon)

Preparation

- In a bowl, combine ground turkey, grated carrots, oats, and turmeric.
- Shape the mixture into meatballs.
- Bake at 350°F (175°C) for 20 minutes or until cooked through.

SALMON AND SWEET POTATO MEDLEY

Ingredients

- Baked salmon flakes (1/2 cup)
- Mashed sweet potatoes (1/4 cup)
- Cooked green beans (1/4 cup)

Preparation

- Combine baked salmon flakes, mashed sweet potatoes, and cooked green beans.
- Mix well and serve at room temperature.

BEEF AND QUINOA STEW

Ingredients

- Lean ground beef (1/2 pound)
- Cooked quinoa (1/2 cup)
- Peas (1/4 cup)
- Parsley (1 tablespoon)

Preparation

- Cook the lean ground beef in a pan until browned.
- Add cooked quinoa, peas, and parsley to the pan.
- Simmer for a few minutes until heated through.
- Allow it to cool before serving.

VEGGIE OMELETTE

Ingredients

- Eggs (2)
- Zucchini (diced) (1/4 cup)
- Spinach (chopped) (1/4 cup)
- Grated cheese (1 tablespoon)

Preparation

- Whisk the eggs in a bowl.
- In a non-stick pan, sauté the diced zucchini and chopped spinach until tender.
- Pour the whisked eggs over the vegetables in the pan.
- Sprinkle grated cheese on top.
- Cook until the omelette is set and the cheese is melted.

- Allow it to cool before serving.

TUNA SALAD SURPRISE

Ingredients

- Canned tuna (in water) (1/4 cup)
- Chopped cucumber (1/4 cup)
- Chopped celery (1/4 cup)
- Plain yogurt (1 tablespoon)

Preparation

- Drain the canned tuna and place it in a bowl.
- Add chopped cucumber, chopped celery, and plain yogurt to the bowl.
- Mix well until all the ingredients are combined.

- Serve chilled.

PUMPKIN AND CARROT SOUP

Ingredients

- Pureed pumpkin (1/2 cup)
- Cooked carrots (mashed) (1/4 cup)
- Low-sodium chicken broth (1/4 cup)

Preparation

- In a saucepan, combine pureed pumpkin, mashed cooked carrots, and low-sodium chicken broth.

- Heat the mixture over medium heat, stirring occasionally, until heated through.

- Allow it to cool slightly before serving.

LENTIL AND VEGETABLE CURRY

Ingredients

- Cooked lentils (1/2 cup)
- Mixed vegetables (such as carrots, peas, and green beans) (1/2 cup)
- Curry powder (1/2 teaspoon)

Preparation

- In a pan, combine cooked lentils, mixed vegetables, and curry powder.
- Cook over medium heat until the vegetables are tender.
- Allow it to cool before serving.

BLUEBERRY BANANA BISCUITS

Ingredients

- Mashed bananas (1/2 cup)
- Blueberries (fresh or frozen) (1/4 cup)
- Whole wheat flour (1 cup)
- Honey (1 tablespoon)

Preparation

- Preheat the oven to 350°F (175°C) and line a baking sheet with parchment paper.
- In a bowl, combine mashed bananas, blueberries, whole wheat flour, and honey.
- Mix until a dough forms.

- Roll out the dough on a lightly floured surface and cut into biscuit shapes.
- Place the biscuits on the prepared baking sheet and bake for 15-20 minutes or until golden brown.
- Allow them to cool completely before serving.

SPINACH AND CHICKEN WRAPS

Ingredients

- Steamed spinach leaves (4-6)
- Cooked chicken breast (sliced) (1/4 cup)

Preparation

- Lay the steamed spinach leaves flat.

- Place sliced cooked chicken breast on top of each leaf.
- Roll the leaves tightly to form wraps.
- Slice the wraps into smaller pieces if desired.
- Serve at room temperature.

BEEF AND SWEET POTATO MEATLOAF

Ingredients

- Lean ground beef (1/2 pound)
- Mashed sweet potatoes (1/2 cup)
- Oats (1/4 cup)
- Grated carrots (1/4 cup)

Preparation

- Preheat the oven to 350°F (175°C) and grease a loaf pan.
- In a bowl, mix together lean ground beef, mashed sweet potatoes, oats, and grated carrots.
- Press the mixture into the greased loaf pan.
- Bake for 30-40 minutes or until cooked through.
- Allow it to cool before serving.

GREEN BEAN AND CHICKEN STIR-FRY

Ingredients

- Sliced chicken breast (cooked) (1/2 cup)
- Green beans (cooked) (1/2 cup)

- Low-sodium soy sauce (1 tablespoon)

Preparation

- In a pan, stir-fry the sliced cooked chicken breast until heated through.
- Add the cooked green beans to the pan and continue stir-frying for a few minutes.
- Pour low-sodium soy sauce over the mixture and stir well.
- Allow it to cool slightly before serving.

APPLE CARROT MUFFINS

Ingredients

- Grated apples (1/2 cup)
- Grated carrots (1/2 cup)

- Whole wheat flour (1 cup)

- Unsweetened applesauce (1/4 cup)

- Preparation:

- Preheat the oven to 350°F (175°C) andline a muffin tin with cupcake liners.

- In a bowl, combine grated apples, grated carrots, whole wheat flour, and unsweetened applesauce.

- Mix until well combined.

- Spoon the batter into the prepared muffin tin, filling each cup about two-thirds full.

- Bake for 20-25 minutes or until a toothpick inserted into the center comes out clean.

- Allow the muffins to cool completely before serving.

SARDINE AND BROWN RICE CASSEROLE

Ingredients

- Canned sardines (in water, drained) (1/2 cup)
- Cooked brown rice (1/2 cup)
- Cooked peas (1/4 cup)
- Dill (1 teaspoon)

Preparation

- Preheat the oven to 350°F (175°C) and grease a casserole dish.
- In the casserole dish, combine canned sardines, cooked brown rice, cooked peas, and dill.
- Mix well.

- Bake for 15-20 minutes or until heated through.
- Allow it to cool slightly before serving.

BROCCOLI AND TURKEY PATTIES

Ingredients

- Chopped broccoli florets (cooked) (1/2 cup)
- Cooked ground turkey (1/2 cup)

Preparation

- In a bowl, combine chopped cooked broccoli florets and cooked ground turkey.
- Mix well.

- Shape the mixture into patties.
- Heat a non-stick pan over medium heat and cook the patties until browned and heated through.
- Allow them to cool before serving.

BERRY BLAST SMOOTHIE

Ingredients

- Blueberries (fresh or frozen) (1/2 cup)
- Strawberries (fresh or frozen) (1/2 cup)
- Plain yogurt (1/4 cup)
- Water (1/4 cup)

Preparation

- In a blender, combine blueberries, strawberries, plain yogurt, and water.

- Blend until smooth and well combined.
- Serve chilled.

QUINOA AND VEGETABLE PILAF

Ingredients

- Cooked quinoa (1/2 cup)
- Mixed vegetables (such as carrots, peas, and green beans) (1/2 cup)
- Olive oil (1 tablespoon)
- Lemon juice (squeeze)

Preparation

- In a pan, heat olive oil over medium heat.

- Add mixed vegetables to the pan and sauté until tender.
- Stir in the cooked quinoa and continue to cook for a few minutes.
- Squeeze lemon juice over the mixture and stir well.
- Allow it to cool before serving.

CHICKEN AND GREEN PEA PASTA

Ingredients

- Cooked pasta (1/2 cup)
- Shredded chicken breast (cooked) (1/4 cup)
- Steamed green peas (1/4 cup)
- Olive oil (1 tablespoon)

Preparation

- In a pan, heat olive oil over medium heat.
- Add cooked pasta, shredded cooked chicken breast, and steamed green peas to the pan.
- Stir well until heated through.
- Allow it to cool slightly before serving.

CARROT AND PARSLEY BISCUITS

Ingredients

- Grated carrots (1/2 cup)
- Fresh parsley (chopped) (1 tablespoon)
- Whole wheat flour (1 cup)

- Beaten egg (1)

Preparation

- Preheat the oven to 350°F (175°C) and line a baking sheet with parchment paper.
- In a bowl, combine grated carrots, chopped fresh parsley, whole wheat flour, and beaten egg.
- Mix until a dough forms.
- Roll out the dough on a lightly floured surface and cut into biscuit shapes.
- Place the biscuits on the prepared baking sheet and bake for 15-20 minutes or until golden brown.
- Allow them to cool completely before serving.

TURKEY AND VEGETABLE STIR-FRY

Ingredients

- Sliced turkey breast (cooked) (1/2 cup)
- Assorted vegetables (such as bell peppers, snap peas, and broccoli) (1 cup)
- Ginger (grated) (1/2 teaspoon)
- Garlic (minced) (1 clove)

Preparation

- In a pan, heat a small amount of olive oil over medium heat.
- Add the sliced cooked turkey breast and stir-fry until heated through.

- Add the assorted vegetables to the pan and continue stir-frying until the vegetables are tender-crisp.
- Stir in the grated ginger and minced garlic and cook for an additional minute.
- Allow it to cool slightly before serving.

MEAL PLAN

DAY 1

Breakfast: Chicken and Rice Delight

Lunch: Turkey Meatballs

Dinner: Salmon and Sweet Potato Medley

DAY 2

Breakfast: Beef and Quinoa Stew

Lunch: Veggie Omelette

Dinner: Tuna Salad Surprise

DAY 3

Breakfast: Pumpkin and Carrot Soup

Lunch: Lentil and Vegetable Curry

Dinner: Blueberry Banana Biscuits

DAY 4

Breakfast: Spinach and Chicken Wraps

Lunch: Beef and Sweet Potato Meatloaf

Dinner: Green Bean and Chicken Stir-Fry

DAY 5

Breakfast: Apple Carrot Muffins

Lunch: Sardine and Brown Rice Casserole

Dinner: Broccoli and Turkey Patties

DAY 6

Breakfast: Berry Blast Smoothie

Lunch: Quinoa and Vegetable Pilaf

Dinner: Chicken and Green Pea Pasta

DAY 7

Breakfast: Carrot and Parsley Biscuits

Lunch: Turkey and Vegetable Stir-Fry

Dinner: Chicken and Rice Delight

CONCLUSION

The power of tested-and-trusted homemade foods shows brightly in the arena of caring for cancer-stricken canines.

These dishes, carefully picked with healthful ingredients and prepared with love, offer a glimmer of hope and support to our four-legged friends fighting this tough disease.

Finding the correct blend of ingredients, flavors, and nutrients can be a daunting task, but the benefits are tremendous.

Homemade recipes that have been tested and trusted provide an opportunity to nourish dogs with meals that are suited to their unique needs, boosting their immune systems and promoting overall well-being.

These recipes have been refined and proven to be beneficial, and they provide a comprehensive approach, incorporating natural proteins, vivid veggies, and antioxidant-rich fruits, all of which are designed to aid in the fight against cancer.

We are reminded of the incredible link we share with our four-legged companions when we see the good impact of these homemade meals.

We provide comfort, care, and a physical display of love with each meal cooked, providing our pets with the sustenance they require to fight their struggle with courage and tenacity.